BREAST CANCER DIET COOKBOOK FOR SENIORS

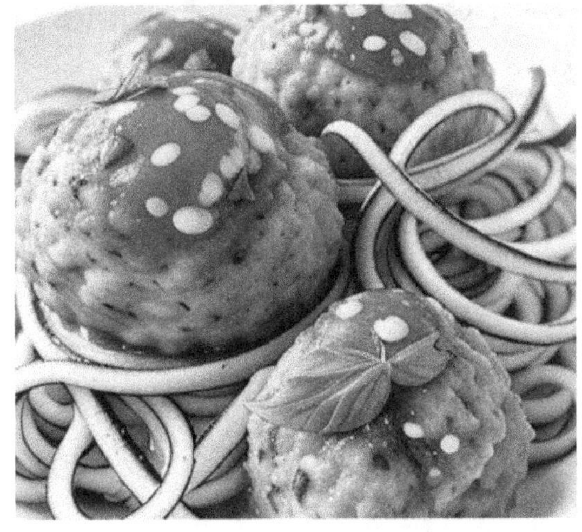

Simple and Delicious Recipes for Fighting Breast Cancer

JESSICA MURRAY

Dear Reader,

Thank you for the purchase. I hope you enjoy and love it, would you consider dropping an honest feedback/review, I will appreciate that and you can contact me using JessicaMurrayDietHelp@gmail.com if you have any questions, I will gladly respond

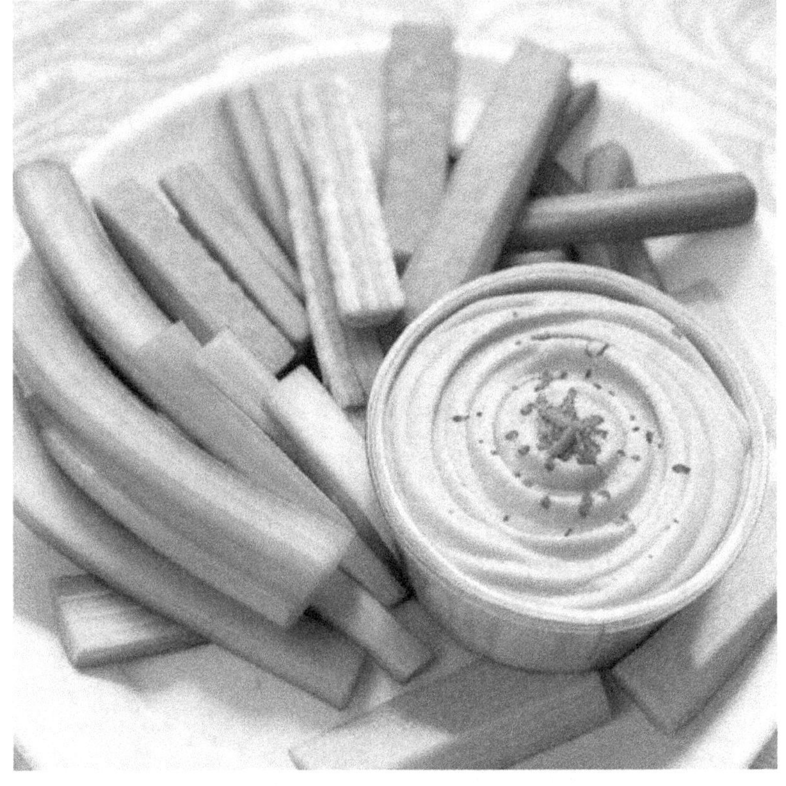

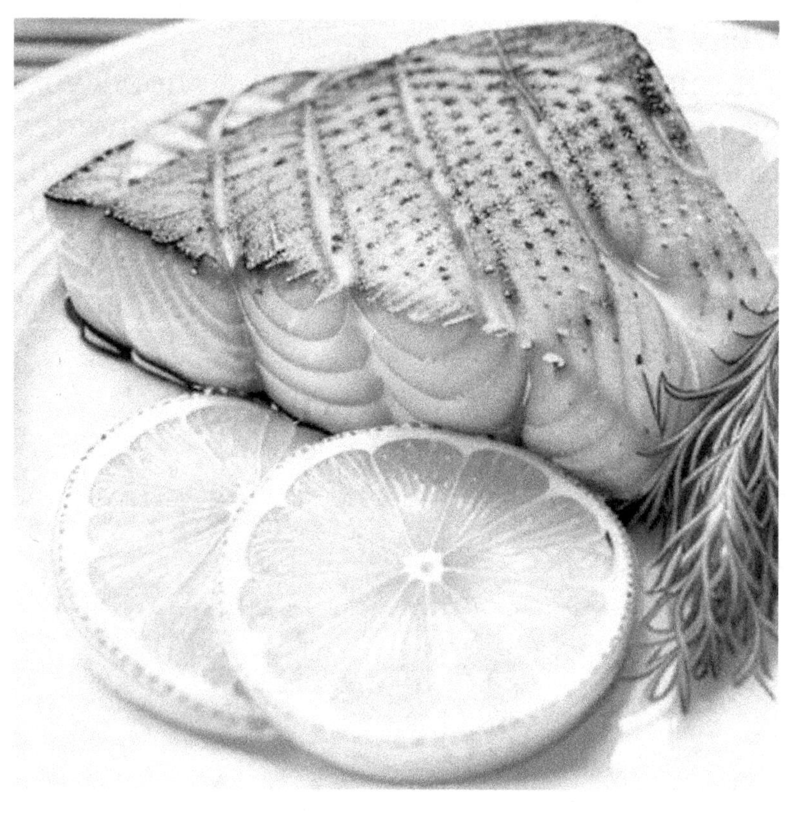

Table of Contents

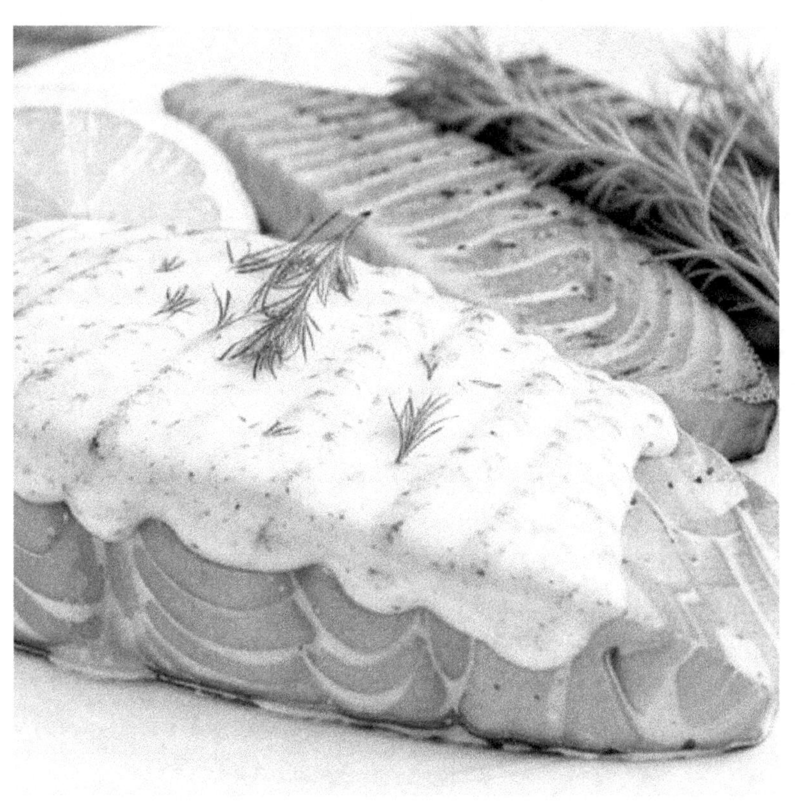

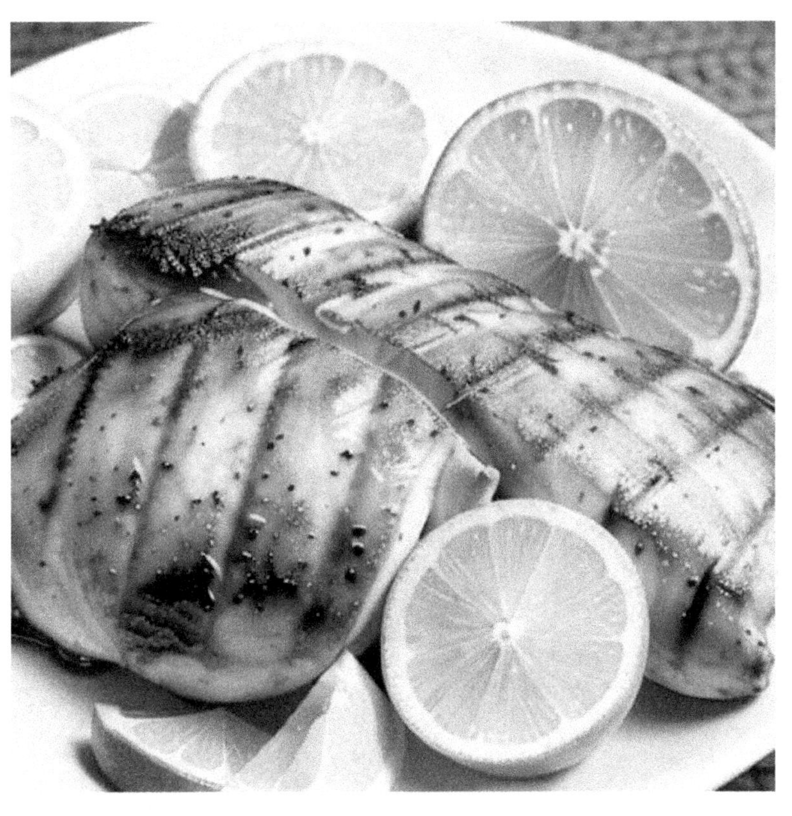

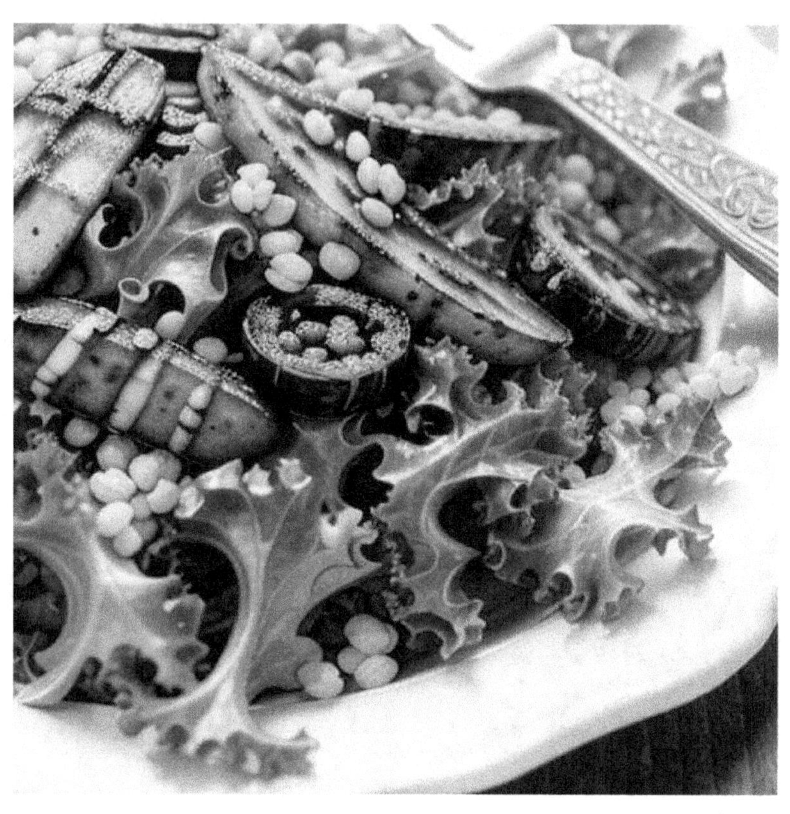

INTRODUCTION

Avibrant senior citizen named Evelyn lived in a thriving suburban community. She was well known in the community for her zest for life and her boisterous laugh. But when she was given the unexpected news that she had breast cancer, her world abruptly changed. Evelyn was ready to take on this challenge despite her first astonishment and apprehension.

Following her diagnosis, Evelyn started looking at different strategies to support her health and wellbeing as she through treatment. She conducted research and discovered the amazing book A Breast Cancer Diet Cookbook for Seniors. The cookbook, written by a prominent nutritionist, included a thorough overview of a diet designed especially for people receiving breast cancer treatment, especially elderly people like Evelyn.

Curiosity piqued, Evelyn dug through the cookbook's pages and found a treasure trove of recipes created to bolster and nourish her body at this important time. The dishes were loaded with nutrient-dense foods, vibrant veggies, and a variety of herbs and spices that are known to have health advantages.

Evelyn set off on her culinary adventure with renewed vigour, equipped with her reliable apron and a shopping list full of colourful ingredients and nutritious food. She devoted her days to experimenting in the kitchen, combining flavours and textures to produce meals that not only delighted her palate but also adhered to the cookbook's dietary suggestions.

As time went on, positive findings from Evelyn's medical exams emerged. Her medical professionals were astounded by the advancements she had made in both her general health and treatment response. Even if the cookbook wasn't a miracle cure, it had unquestionably improved Evelyn's health and complemented the medical treatment she was receiving.

Evelyn's story is one of success and tenacity. Her empowering decisions, such as her choosing to adopt a diet that aided her recovery, were made as she navigated the difficulties of breast cancer. She became an inspiration to everyone going through a similar struggle, not just her peers.

The story of Evelyn thus emphasizes the need of making wise decisions when it comes to our health. Her experience serves as a reminder that, even in the face of hardship, we have the ability to make wise decisions that can result in amazing improvements. Evelyn's spirit remained unwavering throughout her journey, demonstrating that one can actually find their way to a better, healthier future with tenacity, a dash of culinary inventiveness, and a touch of hope.

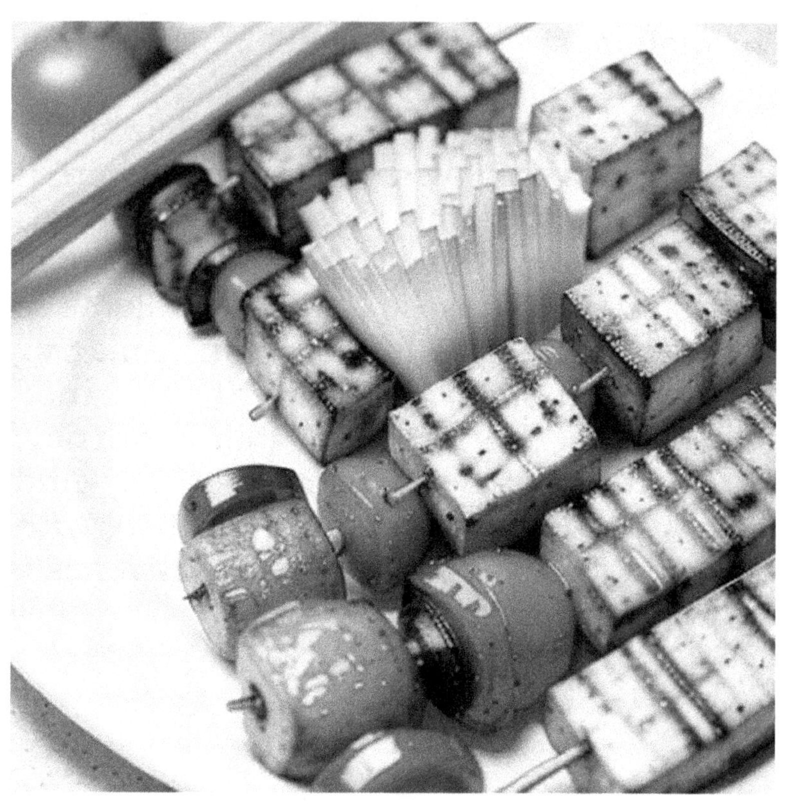

CHAPTER 1

Breakfast Recipes
Chia Seed Pudding with Mixed Berries

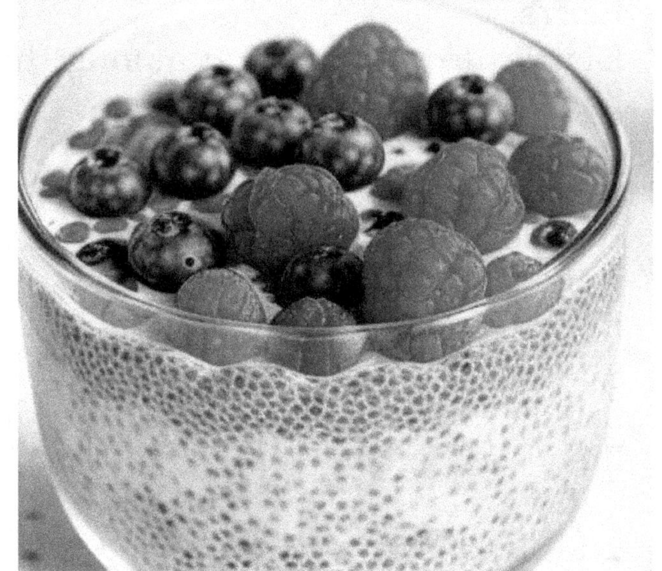

Ingredients:

- 2 cups of almond or coconut milk;
- 1/2 cup of chia seeds.
- 1 cup of mixed berries (raspberries, blueberries, or blackberries) and
- 2 teaspoons of honey

Instructions:

- Mix the milk, chia seeds, and honey in a medium bowl.

- After mixing everything, wait for 15 minutes.
- Include the berries and mix well.
- Put the food in the fridge for up to two hours.
- Distribute the pudding among the 4 bowls, then eat.

Citrus-Marinated Grilled Chicken

Ingredients:

- Boneless, skinless chicken breasts weighing 2 pounds are the ingredients for the citrus-marinated grilled chicken.
- freshly squeezed orange juice and lime juice, each amount equal to 1/4 cup.
- 2 tablespoons olive oil
- 2 minced garlic cloves
- 2 teaspoons of hot sauce
- One teaspoon cumin
- To taste, salt and pepper

Instructions:

- Combine the olive oil, garlic, cumin, chili powder, lime juice, and orange juice in a medium bowl. To blend, stir.

- Add the marinade to the chicken breasts and toss to coat. For at least an hour and up to eight hours, cover and chill.
- Set the grill's temperature to medium-high.
- Take the marinated chicken out of the liquid and sprinkle it with salt and pepper.
- Grill the chicken for 6 to 8 minutes on each side, or until fully done.
- Provide your favourite sides with the chicken.

Cabbage and Carrot Slaw with Light Dressing

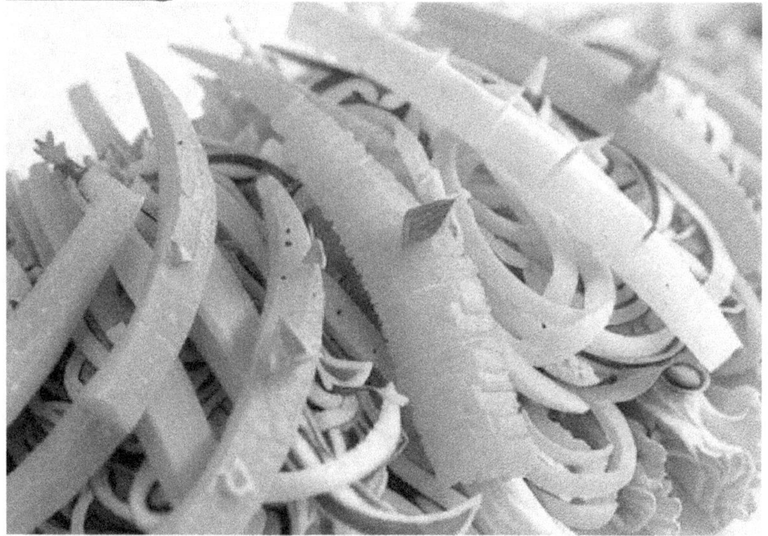

Ingredients:

- 1/2 head of cabbage, finely chopped
- 2 grated carrots;
- 1/4 cup mayonnaise
- 1 tablespoon each of whole-grain mustard;
- 1 tablespoon each of apple cider vinegar;
- 1 tablespoon each of
- Two tablespoons of honey and
- two tablespoons of olive oil should be used.
- To taste, salt and pepper

Instructions:

- Combine the grated carrots and sliced cabbage in a big basin.
- Combine the mayonnaise, mustard, vinegar, and honey in a separate bowl.
- Add the olive oil gradually while whisking the dressing to emulsify it.
- After adding the dressing, mix the cabbage and carrots to coat them thoroughly.
- To taste, add salt and pepper to the food.
- Whether at room temperature or chilled, serve.

Blueberry-Oat Breakfast Muffins

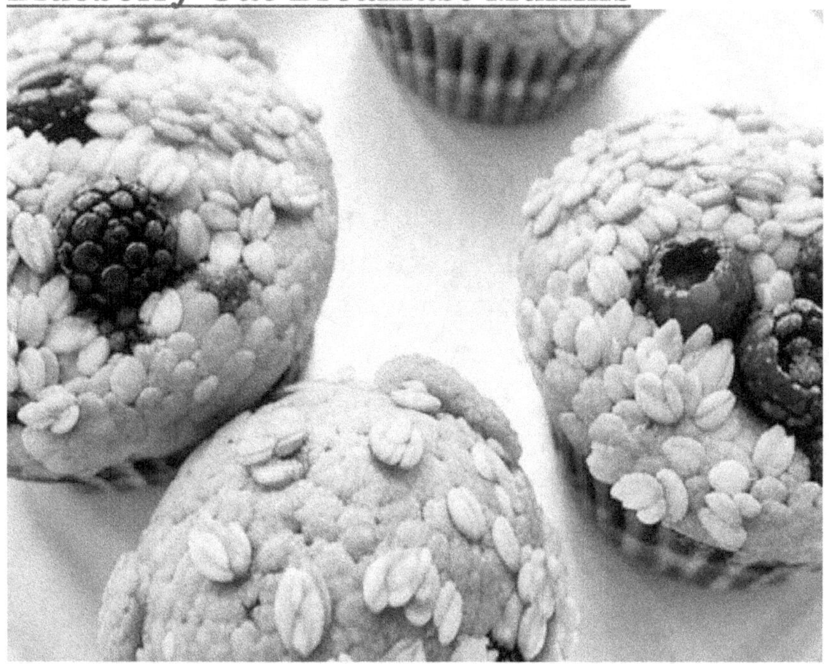

Ingredients:

- 1 teaspoon baking powder and 2 cups of oats
- Baking soda, 1/4 teaspoon
- 1/2 teaspoon of cinnamon, ground
- salt, 1/4 teaspoon
- One cup of Greek yogurt, plain
- honey, 1/4 cup
- 2 eggs
- 1 teaspoon of vanilla essence, 1/4 cup of heated coconut oil, and 1 cup of fresh or frozen blueberries

Instructions:

- Increase the oven's temperature to 350 degrees.
- Use coconut oil to grease a 12-cup muffin tray.
- Combine the oats, baking powder, baking soda, cinnamon, and salt in a medium basin.
- Combine yogurt, honey, eggs, coconut oil, and vanilla extract in another bowl.
- After combining the ingredients with a quick whisk, add the wet elements to the dry mixture.
- Add the blueberries and stir.
- Distribute the batter between the 12 muffin tins.
- Bake the muffins for 20 to 22 minutes, or until a toothpick inserted in the centre comes out clean.
- Transfer to a wire rack after cooling in the pan for five minutes.

Scrambled Egg Tacos with Avocado and Salsa

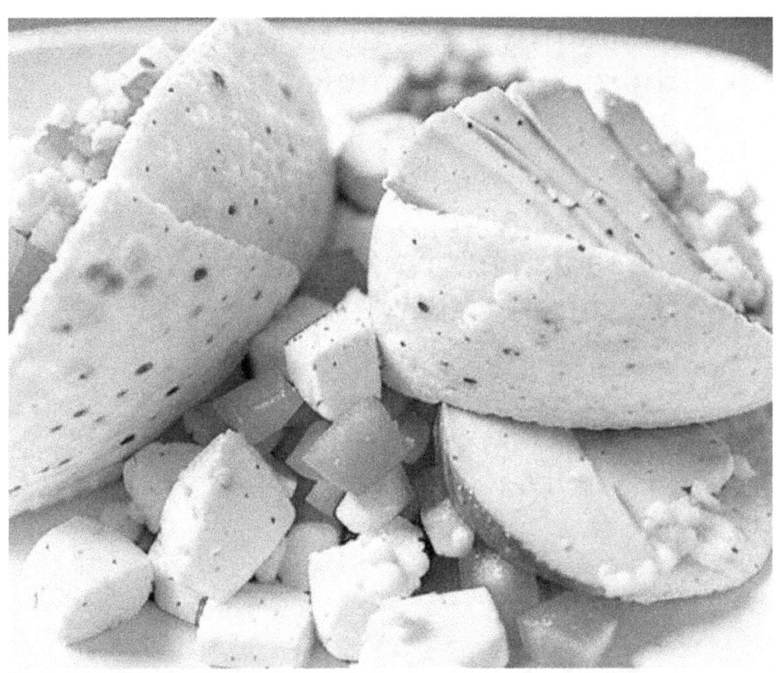

Ingredients:

- 6 eggs and 1 tablespoon of olive oil.
- 1/4 teaspoon each of ground black pepper and salt
- 2 sliced avocados
- One-half cup of salsa
- 6 tortillas, tiny

Instructions:

- In a big skillet over medium heat, warm the olive oil.
- After cracking the eggs, add salt and pepper to the skillet. Cook for approximately 5 minutes, stirring

frequently, or until the eggs are thoroughly scrambled.

- Spread heated tortillas with the scrambled eggs.
- Add salsa and avocado slices to the tacos as garnish.
- Serve right away.

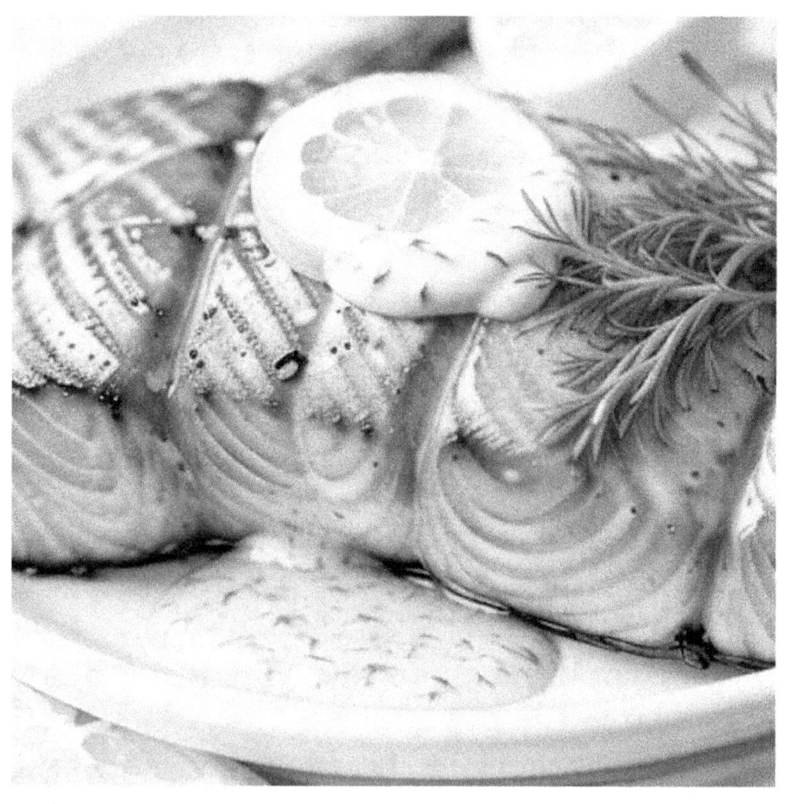

CHAPTER 2

Lunch Recipes

Creamy Broccoli Soup

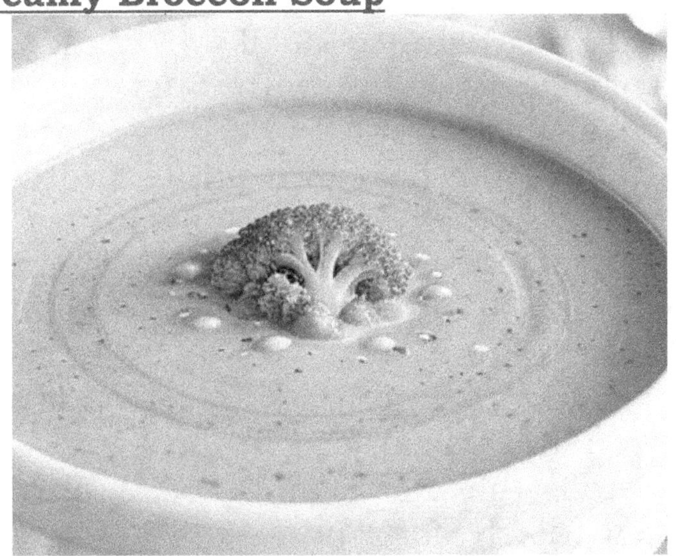

Ingredients:

- 4 cups broccoli florets,
- 4 tablespoons butter,
- 1 chopped onion,
- 2 minced garlic cloves,
- 1/4 cup all-purpose flour,
- 4 cups chicken stock,
- 2 cups milk,
- 1/2 cup grated Parmesan cheese, salt,

- and freshly ground black pepper are the ingredients.

Instructions:
- Fill a big saucepan with broccoli florets. Bring to a boil over high heat, covering them with just enough water to cover.
- Lower the heat to medium and cook the broccoli for 8 to 10 minutes, or until tender. Drain, then set apart.
- Melt the butter over medium heat in the same pan. For 3–4 minutes, or until the onion is softened, add the onion and garlic.
- Add the flour and cook, stirring regularly, for 1 minute.
- Slowly pour in the chicken broth while swirling constantly to avoid lumps.
- Include the milk and simmer over medium heat. Simmer for 8 to 10 minutes while occasionally stirring.
- Include the cooked broccoli in the saucepan and taste-test the seasonings of salt and pepper.
- Puree the soup with an immersion blender until it's smooth.

- Add the Parmesan cheese and taste-
  test the flavour.
- Present hot.

Spinach and Feta Stuffed Portobello Mushrooms

Ingredients:
- 4 big Portobello mushrooms,
- 2 tablespoons olive oil,
- 2 cups baby spinach, 1 minced garlic clove,
- 4 ounces crumbled feta cheese,
- Add 2 teaspoons of freshly chopped parsley to the dish and season generously with salt and freshly ground black pepper.

Instructions:
- Set the oven to 350 degrees.
- Cut off the mushroom stems and lightly oil the underside of the mushrooms. Set in a baking pan.
- Combine the spinach, garlic, feta, and parsley in a small bowl. To taste, add salt and pepper to the food.
- Insert the spinach mixture inside the mushrooms.

- Bake for 20 minutes in a preheated oven, or until the filling is faintly brown and the mushrooms are soft.
- Present hot.

Carrot Soup with Turmeric And Ginger

Ingredients:

- 1 tablespoon olive oil,
- 1 chopped onion,
- 1 tablespoon each of fresh ginger and turmeric,
- 6 cups of vegetable broth,
- 3 cups of peeled and diced carrots,
- 1 tablespoon honey, salt, and freshly ground black pepper.

Instructions:

- In a big pot over medium-high heat, warm the olive oil.
- After the onion has softened, add the ginger and turmeric and simmer for an additional 3 to 4 minutes.
- Include the carrots and vegetable broth, and then bring to a boil. The carrots should be soft after 20 to 25 minutes of simmering at medium-low heat.
- Puree the soup with an immersion blender until it's smooth.

- Add the honey and season to taste with salt and pepper.
- Present hot.

Lentil and Kale Salad with Balsamic Vinaigrette

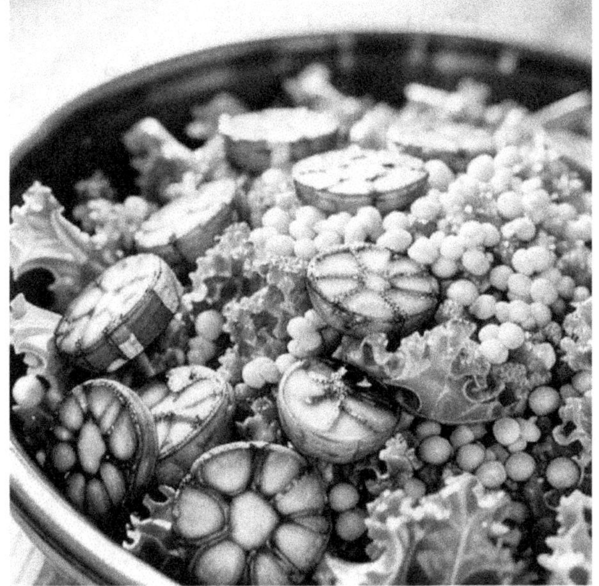

Ingredients:
- 1 cup dry lentils,
- 3 cups chopped kale,
- 1 diced red bell pepper,
- 2 tablespoons diced red onion,
- 1 tablespoon fresh parsley chopped,
- 2 tablespoons balsamic vinegar,
- 2 tablespoons olive oil,

- 1 teaspoon dijon mustard, salt, and freshly ground black pepper.

Instructions:
- Put the lentils in a medium pot in step one.
- Over high heat, add three cups of water and raise the heat until it reaches a full boil.
- Reduce the heat to low and let the lentils simmer covered for 18 to 20 minutes, or until they are cooked through.
- Pour off any extra liquid, then add the lentils to a big bowl.
- Fill the bowl with the kale, bell pepper, onion, and parsley. Combine by tossing.
- Combine the balsamic vinegar, olive oil, and dijon mustard in a small bowl. To taste, add salt and pepper to the food.
- Drizzle the salad with the dressing and toss to mix.
- Serve your food at room temperature.

Baked White Fish with Herbed Quinoa

Ingredients:
- 2 cups cooked quinoa,

- 2 tablespoons chopped fresh parsley, and
- 2 tablespoons chopped fresh thyme.
- 4 6-ounce white fish fillets.
- 2 tablespoons olive oil.
- 2 tablespoons white wine.
- 2 tablespoons fresh lemon juice.

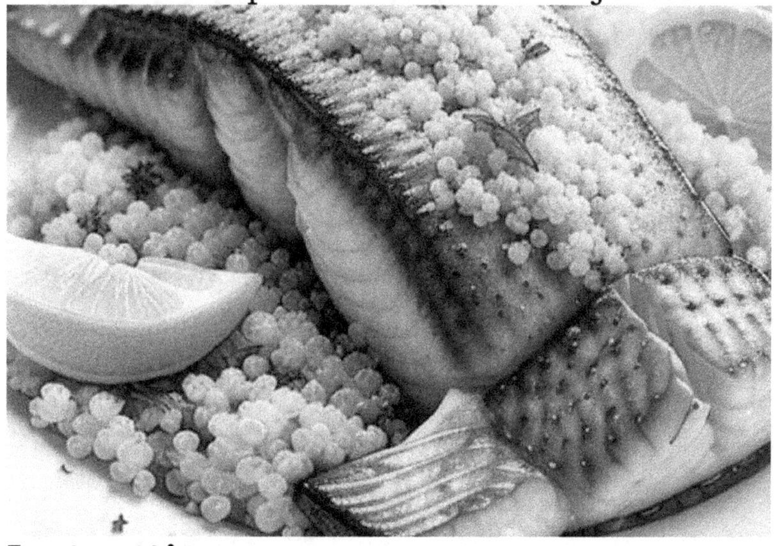

Instructions:

- Set the oven to 400 degrees.
- Rub lemon juice, white wine, and olive oil onto fish fillets.
- After adding the desired amount of salt and black pepper to the desired dish, be sure to taste it to ensure that it meets your expectations.

- Arrange the fillets on a baking sheet and cook them in a preheated oven for 10 to 12 minutes, or until done.
- In the meantime, combine the cooked quinoa, parsley, and thyme in a medium bowl.
- Spoon the quinoa with herbs alongside the fish.

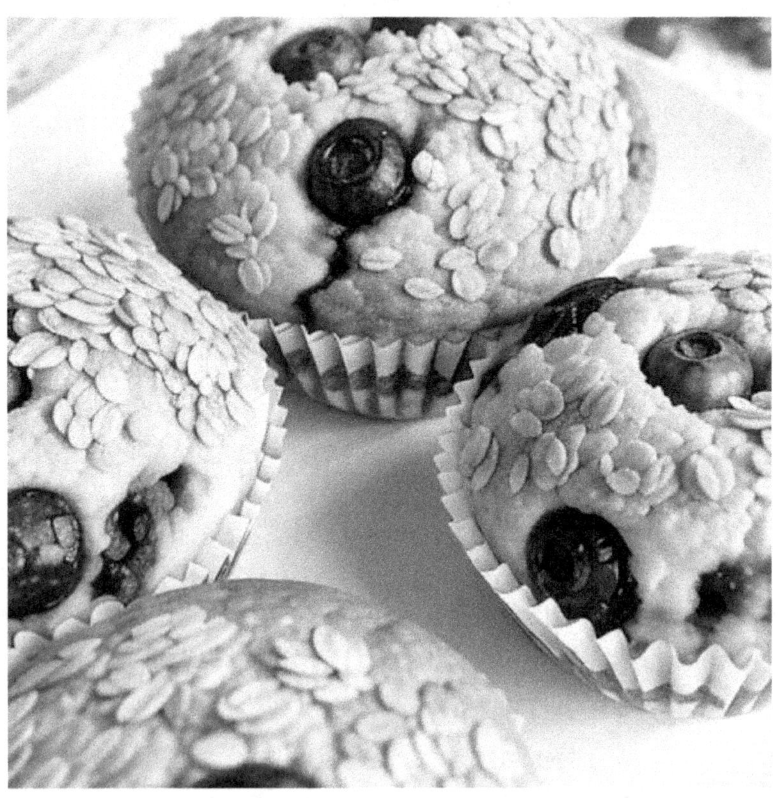

CHAPTER 3

Dinner Recipes
Grilled Salmon with Lemon-Dill Sauce

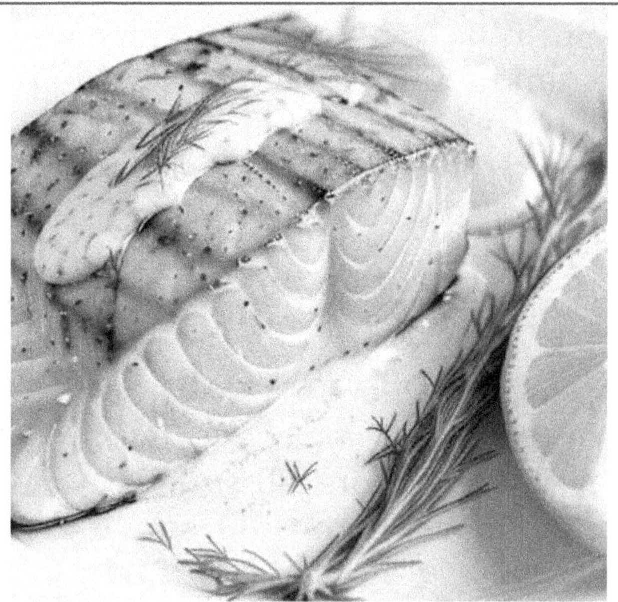

Ingredients:
- 3 tablespoons of olive oil,
- 4 (4-ounce) salmon fillets.
- In order to give your dish the perfect flavouring, add a generous amount of salt and pepper to bring out the pleasing taste of the food.
- In addition to the other ingredients, two tablespoons of lemon juice should also be added.

- 2 teaspoons freshly chopped dill

Instructions:

- Turn the heat to medium-high on a grill or grill pan.
- Sprinkle salt and pepper over the salmon fillets before brushing with olive oil.
- After the grill has been hot, add the fillets and cook them for 3 minutes on each side.
- Combine the lemon juice and dill in a small bowl.
- Cook the fillets for two more minutes on the grill before brushing them with the lemon-dill sauce.
- Add more lemon-dill sauce and hot salmon to the plate.

Roasted Chicken with Garlic and Herbs

Ingredients:

- 2 tablespoons olive oil,
- 2 minced garlic cloves, and
- 4 entire chicken legs.
- One teaspoon of freshly chopped rosemary and
- one teaspoon of freshly chopped thyme.
- To taste, salt and pepper

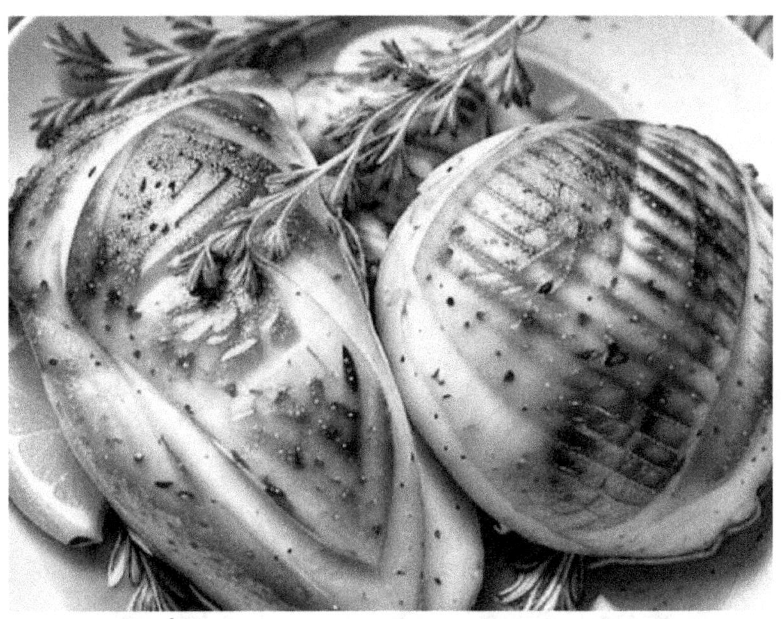

Instructions:

- Set the oven's temperature to 425 F.
- Arrange the chicken legs on an aluminium foil-lined baking sheet.
- Combine the olive oil, garlic, rosemary, thyme, salt, and pepper in a small bowl.
- Combine, then generously brush the mixture over the chicken legs.
- After the oven has been warmed, put the baking sheet inside and roast the chicken for 25 minutes, or until it is thoroughly done.
- Present hot.

Baked Cod with Tomato-Cucumber Salsa

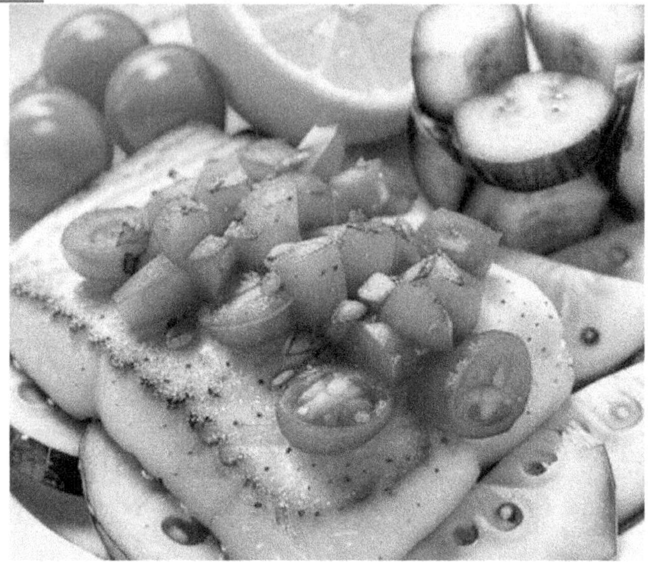

Ingredients:

- 2 tablespoons of olive oil, 4 (6-ounce) cod fillets.
- Two cups of diced tomatoes should be added, and salt and pepper should be added to taste.
- 1 cup cucumbers, diced
- 2 tablespoons fresh cilantro that has been chopped,
- 2 tablespoons olive oil, and
- 2 tablespoons lime juice.

Instructions:

- Set the oven's temperature to be 400 degrees Fahrenheit.
- Arrange the fish fillets on an aluminium foil-lined baking sheet.
- Sprinkle salt and pepper over the fillets after brushing them with olive oil.
- Combine the tomatoes, cucumber, cilantro, olive oil, and lime juice in a medium bowl.
- After the oven has been prepared, put the baking sheet inside and bake the fish for 20 minutes, or until it is thoroughly done.
- Spoon tomato-cucumber salsa on top of the heated cod.

Herbed Turkey Meatballs with Zucchini Noodles

Ingredients:

- 1 pound minced garlic and
- 2 minced cloves of minced fresh parsley.
- 1 tsp. dried oregano
- One-half of a teaspoon of dried thyme.
- 2 tablespoons of extra virgin olive oil,

- 2 medium spiralized zucchini, salt, and pepper to taste

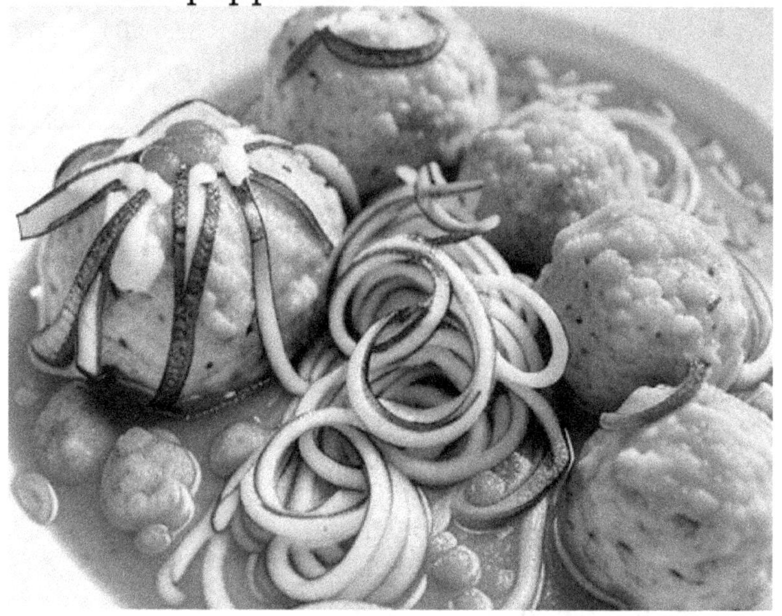

Instructions:

- In order to prepare the food properly, the oven needs to be set to a temperature of 400 degrees Fahrenheit.
- Combine the ground turkey, parsley, garlic, oregano, thyme, salt, and pepper in a sizable bowl.
- Shape the ingredients into 12 meatballs of the same size.
- Arrange the meatballs on an aluminium foil-lined baking sheet.

- Bake the meatballs for 20 minutes, or until they are well heated through.
- In the meantime, warm up a big skillet with olive oil over medium heat.
- After adding, simmer the zucchini noodles for 3 minutes, or until they are soft.
- Combine the hot zucchini noodles with the turkey meatballs.

Grilled Tofu and Vegetable Skewers

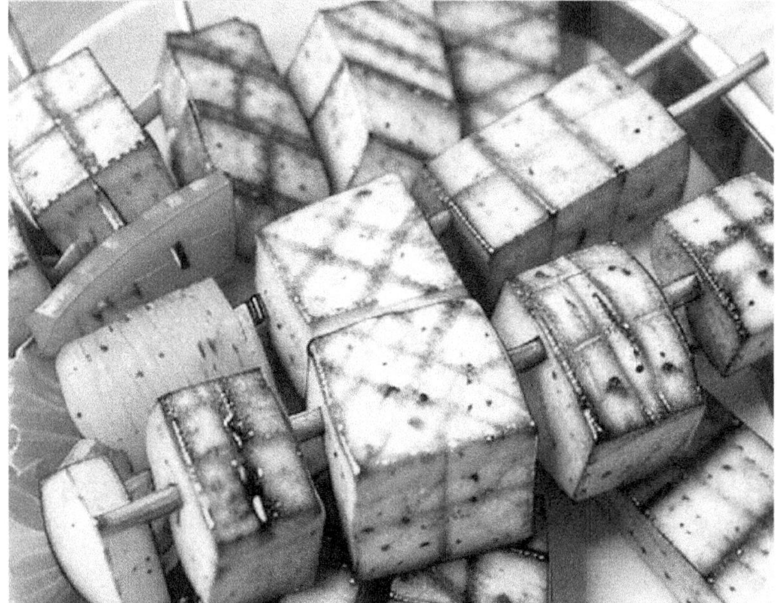

Ingredients:

- 1 (14 ounce) block extra-firm tofu that has been cubed,

- 1 red bell pepper that has been seeded and chopped,
- 1 yellow bell pepper that has been seeded and chopped, and
- 1 red onion that has been cubed.
- Olive oil, 2 tablespoons
- 2 teaspoons soy sauce
- 2 minced garlic cloves
- fresh ginger, 1 teaspoon
- To taste, salt and pepper

Instructions:

- Turn the heat to medium-high on the grill or grill pan.
- Alternately thread the tofu, bell peppers, and onion onto metal skewers.
- Combine the olive oil, soy sauce, garlic, ginger, salt, and pepper in a small bowl.
- Liberally brush the marinade on the skewers.
- Cook the skewers on the grill for 4 minutes on each side, or until the vegetables are cooked.
- Present hot.

CHAPTER 4

Snacks and Desserts

Roasted Chickpea Crunchies

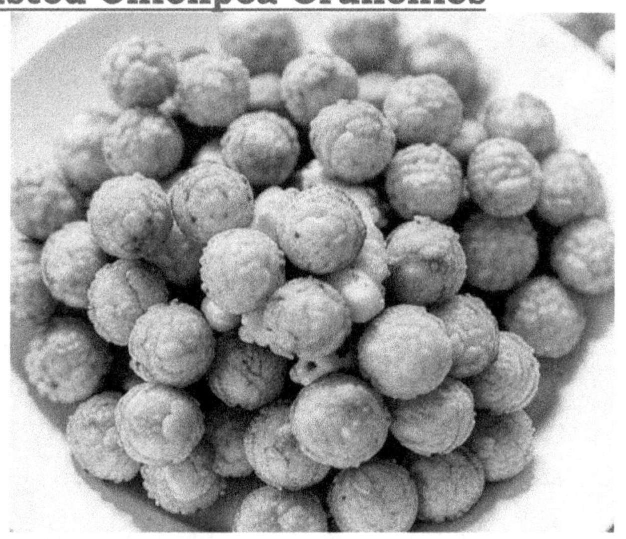

Ingredients:

- 2 cans of chickpeas,
- 2 tablespoons of extra virgin olive oil, 1 teaspoon each of garlic powder, smoked paprika, cumin, onion powder, and oregano, as
- In addition to the ingredients previously mentioned, one should also add salt and black pepper to taste.

Instructions:

- Set the oven to 400 °F. Before patting the chickpeas dry with a paper towel, drain and rinse them. Add olive oil, cumin, onion powder, oregano, smoked paprika, garlic powder, salt, and pepper to the large bowl of chickpeas. Stir everything together until the spices are equally distributed over the chickpeas.
- For optimal results, spread the chickpeas in a single layer on a baking sheet that has been lined with parchment paper. This will help ensure that they cook evenly and that they don't stick to the pan.
- Cook the chickpeas in the oven for 30 minutes, stirring regularly, or until they are crisp and golden brown. Serve right away.

Chia Pudding Delight

Ingredients:

- 2 cups almond milk,
- 1 cup chia seeds,
- 2 tablespoons maple syrup,
- 1 teaspoon vanilla essence,
- 2 teaspoons ground cinnamon, and
- 1 cup chopped walnuts.

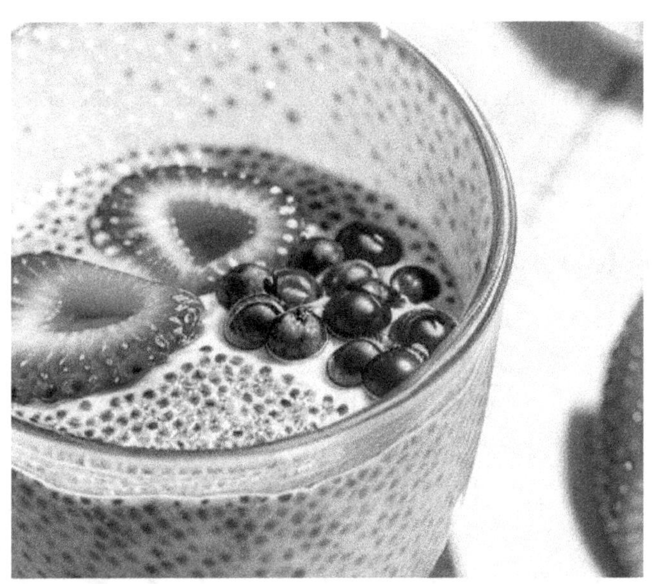

Instructions:

- Assemble the ingredients in a medium bowl by stirring the chia seeds, almond milk, maple syrup, vanilla essence, and ground cinnamon until well-combined.
- Stir the mixture occasionally while letting it sit for 15 minutes. Put the pudding on a serving dish and sprinkle chopped walnuts on top.
- Serve after one hour in the refrigerator.

Almond Butter Apple Slices

Ingredients:

- two tiny apples, two teaspoons of almond butter, two tablespoons of unsweetened shredded coconut, two tablespoons of chia seeds, and one tablespoon of honey.

Instructions:

- Spread out the apple wedges on a platter after thinly slicing them. On top of the apples, drizzle the almond butter, coconut shavings, and chia seeds.
- Honey should be drizzled on top before serving.

Veggie Sticks with Hummus

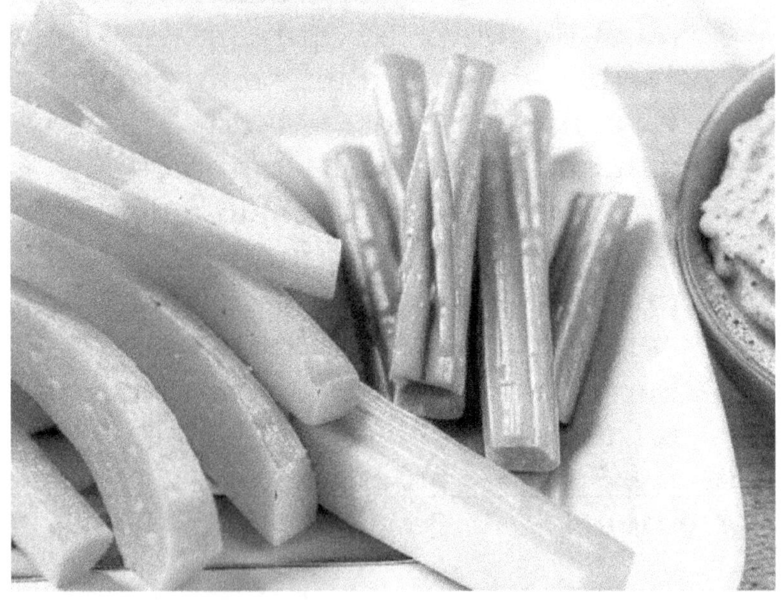

Ingredients:

- 2 carrot sticks,
- 2 celery sticks, and
- 1/2 cup hummus

Ingredients:

- Put the carrots and celery sticks in a serving bowl with the hummus.

Quinoa Berry Bars

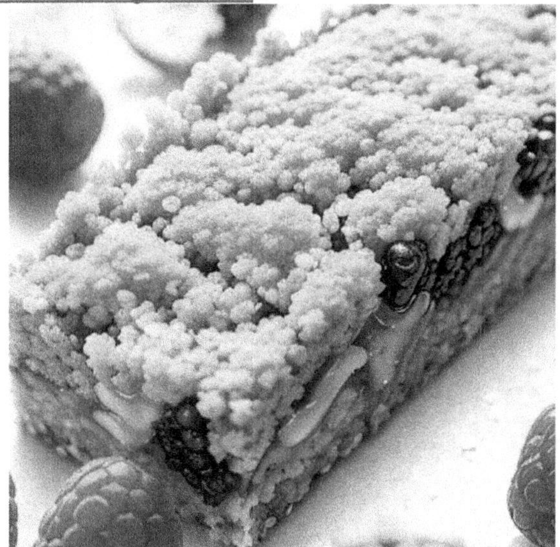

Ingredients:

- 1 cup cooked quinoa, a half cup of almond flour,
- a half teaspoon of baking powder, three tablespoons of coconut oil,
- two mashed bananas, a tablespoon of honey,

- a teaspoon of vanilla essence,
- and a cup of frozen mixed berries

Instructions:

- Set the oven to 350°F.
- Combine the cooked quinoa, almond flour, and baking powder in a sizable basin.
- Combine the coconut oil, mashed banana, honey, and vanilla extract in another bowl.
- Stir the quinoa mixture while adding the wet components to ensure that everything is well-combined.
- Add the frozen mixed berries by blending.
- Spread the quinoa mixture evenly over the parchment paper-lined 8x8 baking sheet.
- For 25 minutes, bake. Just before slicing and serving, let the pan cool.

Dark Chocolate Avocado Mousse

Ingredients:

- 2 avocados,
- 1/4 cup chocolate powder,
- 1/4 cup maple syrup, and
- a dash of vanilla.

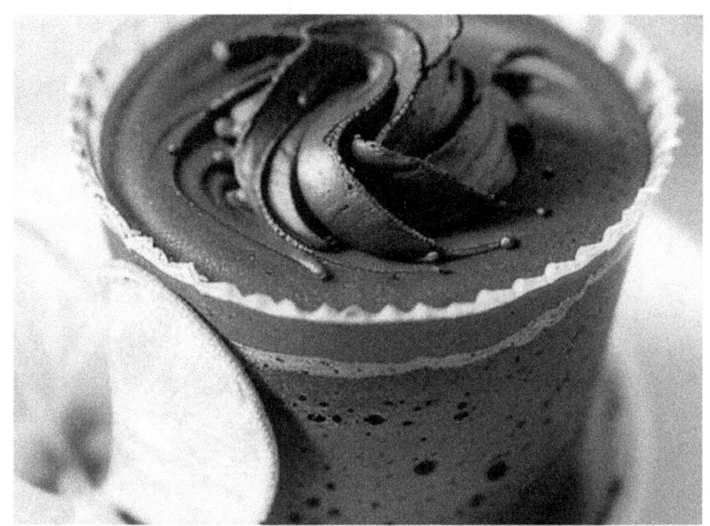

Instructions:

- The avocados should be peeled, pitted, and added to a food processor.
- Blend in the cocoa powder, maple syrup, and vanilla extract until the mixture has a smooth texture.
- Before serving, place the mousse in small serving bowls and chill for an hour.

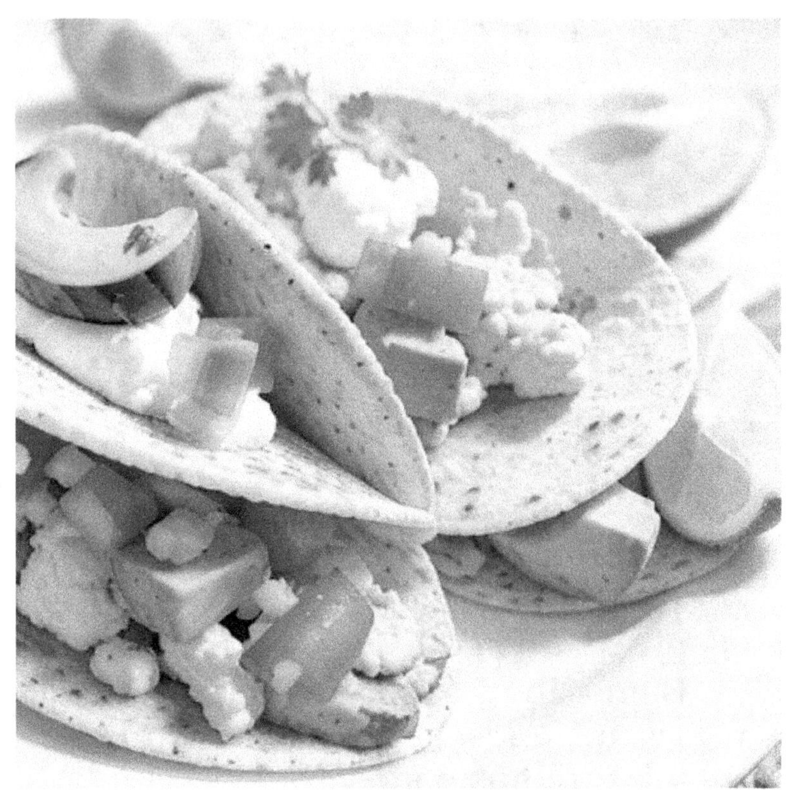

CHAPTER 5

Smoothies and Juicing

Berry Bliss Antioxidant Blend

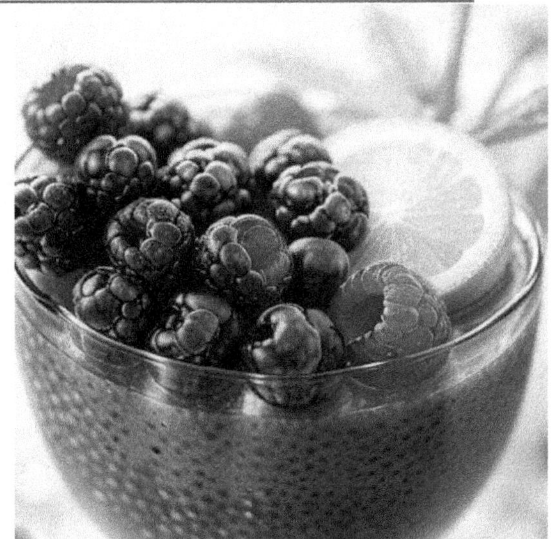

Ingredients:

- 1/2 cup strawberries, frozen
- 1/2 cup blueberries, frozen
- 1/2 cup blackberries, frozen
- 1 banana, ripe
- half a cup of almond milk
- one spoonful of honey

Instructions:

- Place all of the ingredients in a blender, and blend until completely smooth.

- If necessary, increase the amount of honey to adjust the sweetness.
- Dish out!

Green Healing Elixir

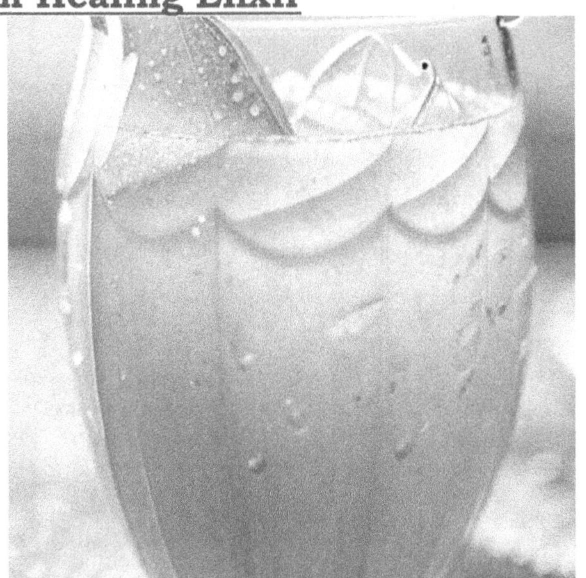

Ingredients:
- 2 bananas and 1 cup of spinach
- 1/2 apple
- half a cup of pineapple
- fresh mint leaves, 1/4 cup
- fresh ginger root, 1/4 cup
- 1/2 lime
- two cups of water

Instructions:

- Put all the ingredients into a blender, and blend until the mixture is completely smooth and consistent.
- If desired, strain the mixture.
- Dish out and savour!

Turmeric Mango Immunity Boost

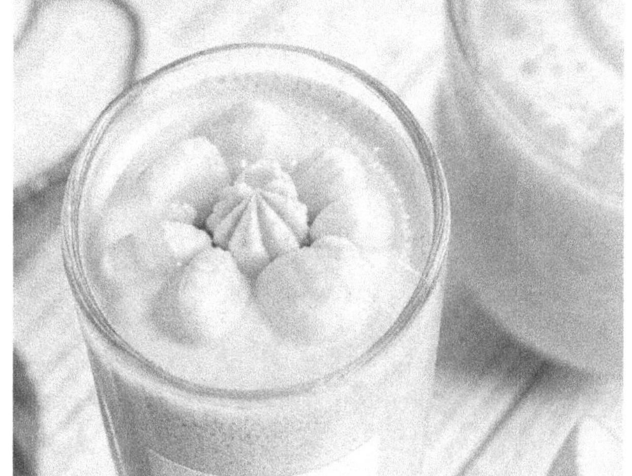

Ingredients:
- a one cup of frozen mango chunks
- 1/four teaspoon of ground turmeric
- 1 cup of unsweetened almond milk and 1/2 teaspoon of honey

Instructions:
- Place all the ingredients in a blender, and process until completely smooth.
- If necessary, increase the amount of honey to adjust the sweetness.
- Dish out

Spinach Berry Revitalize Smoothie

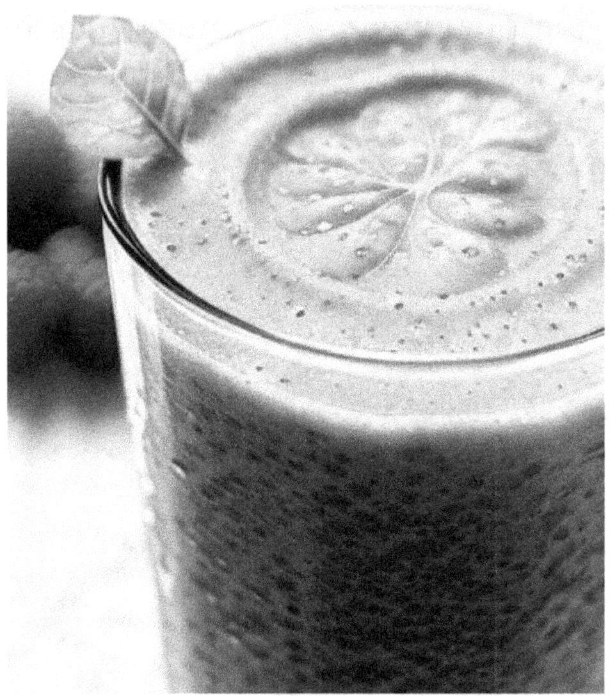

Ingredients:

- 1/2 cup frozen strawberries and
- 1 cup frozen spinach.
- 1/2 cup blueberries, frozen
- half a cup of almond milk
- one spoonful of honey

Instructions:

- Place all the ingredients in a blender, and process until thoroughly combined.

- If necessary, increase the amount of honey to adjust the sweetness.
- Savour!

Blueberry Kale Power Punch

Ingredients:

- 1/2 cup frozen blueberries
- 2-cups of kale
- 1/2 cup almond milk without added sugar
- one spoonful of honey

Instructions:

- Place all the ingredients in a blender, and process until completely smooth.
- If necessary, increase the amount of honey to adjust the sweetness.
- Dish out

Beetroot Berry Detox Blend

Ingredients:

- 1/2 cup frozen strawberries are among the ingredients.
- 1/2 cup blueberries, frozen
- fresh beetroot, 1/2 cup
- 1/2 cup almond milk without added sugar
- one spoonful of honey

Instructions:

- Place all the ingredients in a blender, and process until completely smooth.
- If necessary, increase the amount of honey to adjust the sweetness.
- savour!

Papaya Carrot Nourishing Juice

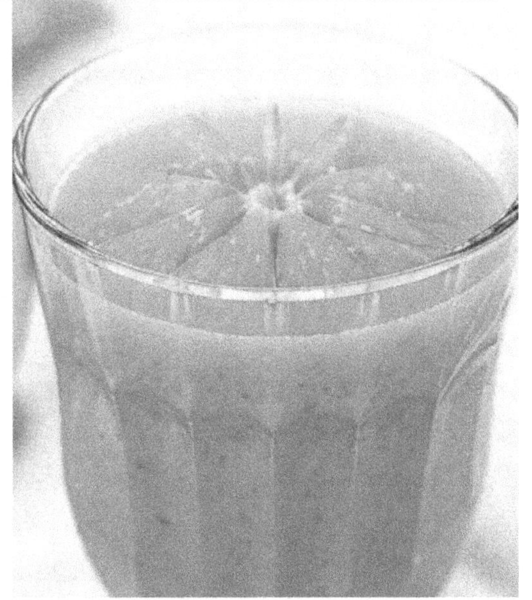

Ingredients:
- 1/2 cup carrot juice and
- 1/2 ripe papaya
- 1.5 cups of water

Instructions:
- Place all the ingredients in a blender, and process until completely smooth.
- Dish out and savor!

CHAPTER 6

7-Day Meal Plan
DAY 1

Breakfast	Lunch	Dinner
Cabbage and Carrot Slaw with Light Dressing	Spinach and Feta Stuffed Portobello Mushrooms	Baked Cod with Tomato-Cucumber Salsa

DAY 2

Breakfast	Lunch	Dinner
Blueberry-Oat Breakfast Muffins	Creamy Broccoli Soup	Grilled Tofu and Vegetable Skewers

DAY 3

Breakfast	Lunch	Dinner
Chia Seed Pudding with Mixed Berries	Carrot Soup with Turmeric And Ginger	Herbed Turkey Meatballs with Zucchini Noodles

DAY 4

Breakfast	Lunch	Dinner
Scrambled Egg Tacos with Avocado and Salsa	Lentil and Kale Salad with Balsamic Vinaigrette	Roasted Chicken with Garlic and Herbs

DAY 5

Breakfast	Lunch	Dinner
Citrus-Marinated Grilled Chicken	Baked White Fish with Herbed Quinoa	Grilled Salmon with Lemon-Dill Sauce

DAY 6

Breakfast	Lunch	Dinner
Blueberry-Oat Breakfast Muffins	Lentil and Kale Salad with Balsamic Vinaigrette	Grilled Tofu and Vegetable Skewers

DAY 7

Breakfast	Lunch	Dinner
Chia Seed Pudding with Mixed Berries	Carrot Soup with Turmeric And Ginger	Roasted Chicken with Garlic and Herbs

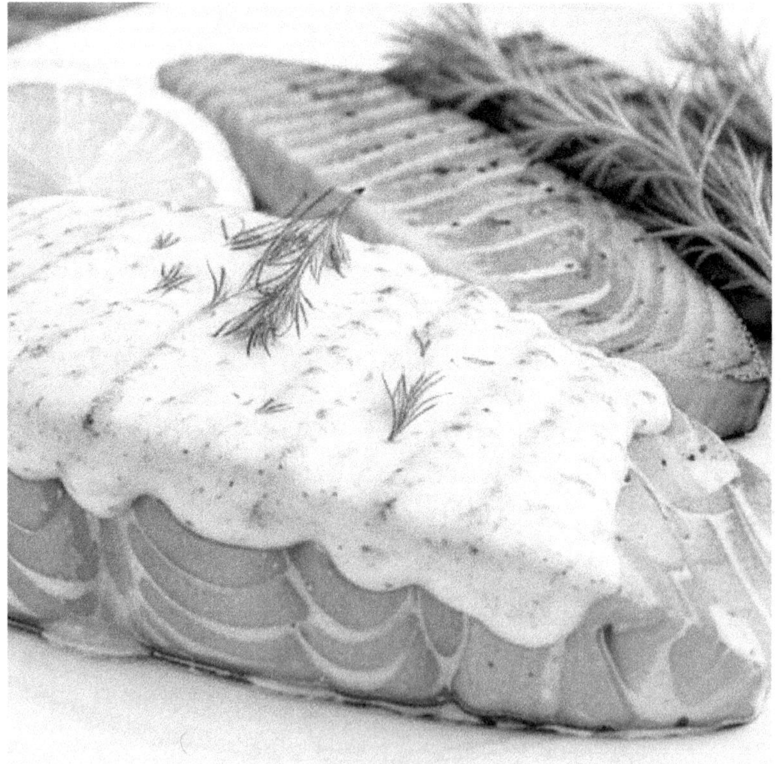

CONCLUSION

As the "Breast Cancer Diet Cookbook for Seniors" draws to an end, it is without a doubt clear that nourishing one's body and soul via thoughtful dietary choices can have a substantial impact on one's journey through and beyond breast cancer. This cookbook serves as an inspiration for senior citizens to embrace a culinary route that promotes their wellbeing.

In these pages, we've shown how nutrition has a significant impact on reducing risks and promoting recovery. We've also shown how delicious taste combinations may be used to transform every meal into a celebration of life. Seniors take control of their health in the most delicious way as they set out on this culinary expedition, armed with knowledge and a bounty of recipes catered to their requirements.

May the dishes in this cookbook serve as a source of inspiration and nurturing, demonstrating how each thoughtful bite is a step toward vitality. Let the overriding lesson in this conclusion be that while age may add years, it is the wisdom in

choosing nourishment that truly adds
years to life.

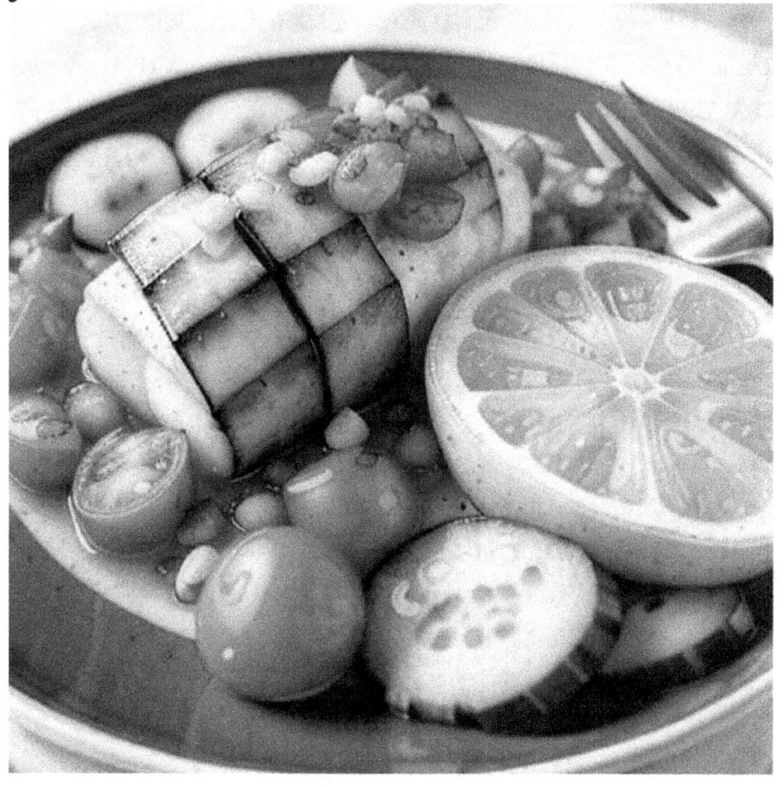

I'm grateful that you took the time to read my book. I hope you like it and it gave you something to think about. Thank You

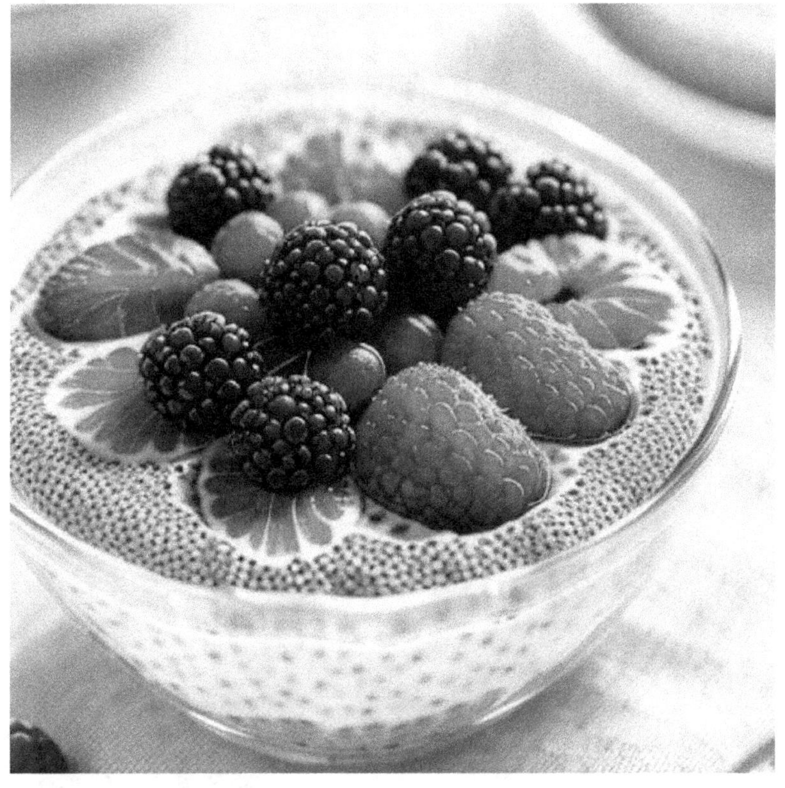

Weekly Meal Planner

KEY

B-Breakfast
L-Lunch
D-Dinner

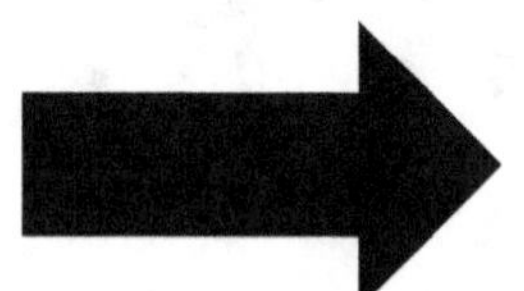

MONDAY	B
	L
	D
TUESDAY	B
	L
	D
WENESDAY	B
	L
	D
THURSDAY	B
	L
	D
FRIDAY	B
	L
	D
SATURDAY	B
	L
	D
SUNDAY	B
	L
	D

MONDAY	B	
	L	
	D	
TUESDAY	B	
	L	
	D	
WENESDAY	B	
	L	
	D	
THURSDAY	B	
	L	
	D	
FRIDAY	B	
	L	
	D	
SATURDAY	B	
	L	
	D	
SUNDAY	B	
	L	
	D	

MONDAY	B
	L
	D
TUESDAY	**B**
	L
	D
WENESDAY	**B**
	L
	D
THURSDAY	**B**
	L
	D
FRIDAY	**B**
	L
	D
SATURDAY	**B**
	L
	D
SUNDAY	**B**
	L
	D

MONDAY	B
	L
	D

TUESDAY	B
	L
	D

WENESDAY	B
	L
	D

THURSDAY	B
	L
	D

FRIDAY	B
	L
	D

SATURDAY	B
	L
	D

SUNDAY	B
	L
	D

MONDAY	B
	L
	D

TUESDAY	B
	L
	D

WENESDAY	B
	L
	D

THURSDAY	B
	L
	D

FRIDAY	B
	L
	D

SATURDAY	B
	L
	D

SUNDAY	B
	L
	D

MONDAY	B
	L
	D

TUESDAY	B
	L
	D

WENESDAY	B
	L
	D

THURSDAY	B
	L
	D

FRIDAY	B
	L
	D

SATURDAY	B
	L
	D

SUNDAY	B
	L
	D

MONDAY	B
	L
	D

TUESDAY	**B**
	L
	D

WENESDAY	**B**
	L
	D

THURSDAY	**B**
	L
	D

FRIDAY	**B**
	L
	D

SATURDAY	**B**
	L
	D

SUNDAY	**B**
	L
	D

DAILY MEAL PLANNER

TO DO	
1	
2	
3	
4	
5	
6	
7	
8	
9	
10	

EXERCISE

GOAL ACTIVITIES

	☐
	☐
	☐
	☐
	☐
	☐
	☐

SHOPPING

<table>
<tr><td colspan="2" align="center">MEALS</td></tr>
<tr><td>BREAKFAST</td><td></td></tr>
<tr><td>LUNCH</td><td></td></tr>
<tr><td>DINNER</td><td></td></tr>
<tr><td>SNACKS</td><td></td></tr>
<tr><td>DESSERTS</td><td></td></tr>
</table>

OBSERVATION

INSPIRATION

NOTES & TIPS

DAILY MEAL PLANNER

TO DO

1	
2	
3	
4	
5	
6	
7	
8	
9	
10	

EXERCISE

GOAL ACTIVITIES

- ☐
- ☐
- ☐
- ☐
- ☐
- ☐
- ☐

SHOPPING

<table>
<tr><td colspan="2">MEALS</td><td>OBSERVATION</td></tr>
<tr><td>BREAKFAST</td><td></td><td></td></tr>
<tr><td>LUNCH</td><td></td><td></td></tr>
<tr><td>DINNER</td><td></td><td></td></tr>
<tr><td>SNACKS</td><td></td><td>INSPIRATION</td></tr>
<tr><td>DESSERTS</td><td></td><td></td></tr>
</table>

NOTES & TIPS

DAILY MEAL PLANNER

TO DO	
1	
2	
3	
4	
5	
6	
7	
8	
9	
10	

EXERCISE

GOAL ACTIVITIES

- ☐
- ☐
- ☐
- ☐
- ☐
- ☐
- ☐

SHOPPING

<table>
<tr><td colspan="2">

MEALS

</td><td>

OBSERVATION

</td></tr>
<tr><td>**BREAKFAST**</td><td></td><td></td></tr>
<tr><td>**LUNCH**</td><td></td><td></td></tr>
<tr><td>**DINNER**</td><td></td><td></td></tr>
<tr><td>**SNACKS**</td><td></td><td>

INSPIRATION

</td></tr>
<tr><td>**DESSERTS**</td><td></td><td></td></tr>
</table>

NOTES & TIPS

www.ingramcontent.com/pod-product-compliance
Lightning Source LLC
Chambersburg PA
CBHW050850260726
48660CB00006B/2545